Introduction To
TRADITIONAL CHINESE MEDICINE

Introduction To
Traditional Chinese Medicine"

Benita and Jim Babeckis

Published for:
TRANZFORMATIONS
Oro Valley, Az. 85704

Email: Tranzform@Comcast.net
Website: http:// Tranzformations.net

Published for Tranzformations
8571 N. Calle Tioga
Oro Valley, Arizona 85704

ISBN No. 978-1440424588

Type composition and design by Full Moon Rising.
Cover illustration by Jim Babeckis - Graphic Design and Illustration. Copyright © 2007. Cover design by Full Moon Rising

First Published October, 2008

Manufactured in the United States of America

Contents

Contents

Introduction

Traditional Chinese medicine (TCM) is an ancient medical system that takes a deep understanding of the laws and patterns of nature and applies them to the human body. TCM is not "New Age," nor is it a patchwork of different healing modalities. TCM is a complete medical system that has been practiced for more than five thousand years.

Chinese medicine is not based on the typical ideas and facts that you would see in every day doctor's offices. The science of Chinese medicine is based on philosophies of the spiritual being in tune to the mental and physical bodies. When all three of these are aligned, it allows for Qi, or energy, to move through your body without any trouble.

If you are looking for your own method of using Chinese medicine, there are several approaches you can take.

There are typically eight different methods of Chinese medicine that are used for healing. Each of these methods can be used simultaneously with others, depending on a person's Qi and what they need. Unlike Western medicine, none of these methods are invasive and have very low side effects. This means that you can try a variety of them on your own and find ones that work best for you.

The first type or category of methods that are used in Chinese medicine are self-administered methods. These are done by someone researching what they need and finding the necessary solutions.

Meditation is a common method that can be used by anyone in order to facilitate healing. Practicing exercises with Qigong, an ancient form to move energy is also common. Exercise and changing your diet to balance out nutrition in a different form is also used as a self-administered method.

If you still are having trouble healing, you can use the second category of methods in order to get the proper alignment. These are the types of healing that are administered by a practitioner who has studied Chinese Medicine.

At the heart of TCM is the tenet that the root cause of illnesses, not their symptoms, must be treated. In modern-day terms, TCM is holistic in its approach; it views every aspect of a person—body, mind, spirit, and emotions—as part of one complete circle rather than loosely connected pieces to be treated individually.

The following is a brief introduction to some of the key terms and concepts in traditional Chinese medicine. It is not meant to be all inclusive.

Often Western CAM practitioners and their patients or clients derive their understanding of TCM from acupuncture. However, acupuncture is only one of the major treatment modalities of this comprehensive medical system based on the understanding of Qi or vital energy.

These major treatment modalities are:

* Qigong: an energy practice, generally encompassing simple movements and postures. Some Qigong systems also emphasize breathing techniques.

* Herbal Therapy: the use of herbal combinations or formulas to strengthen and support organ system function.

* Acupuncture: the insertion of needles in "acupoints" to help Qi flow smoothly.

* Acupressure: the use of specific hand techniques to help Qi flow smoothly.

* Foods for Healing: the prescription of certain foods for healing based on their energy essences or energy signatures, not nutritional value.

* Chinese Psychology: the understanding of emotions and their relationship to the internal organ systems and their influence on health.

The Theory of Qi (Chi)

The true foundation of TCM is Qi, which is loosely translated as vital energy. In TCM, Qi is considered to be the force that animates and informs all things. In the human body, Qi flows through meridians, or energy pathways. Twelve major meridians run through the body, and it is over this network that Qi travels through the body and that the body's various organs send messages to one another.

For this reason, keeping the meridians clear is imperative for the body's self-regulating actions to occur. Through proper training, people can develop the sensitivity to feel the flow of Qi.

While it is often described in the West as energy, or vital energy, the term Qi carries a deeper meaning. Qi has two aspects: one is energy, power, or force; the other is conscious intelligence or information.

Each Organ System carries its own unique Qi, which allows it to perform its unique functions —both physical (which Western medicine can describe) and energetic (which Eastern medicine can identify). This energetic function also includes an Organ System's relationship with other organs. (Organ is here capitalized to distinguish the TCM concept of an Organ System and its functions from the Western concept of the physical organ.)

TCM frequently references several major Qi, or energy function, problems. One is an overall "Qi deficiency," which is often described in Western medical terms as chronic fatigue syndrome (CFS). TCM also has the knowledge and ability to pinpoint which Organs have an energy deficiency. Another major condition is described as "Qi stagnation," which means energy and information cannot move smoothly to or from its appropriate location. For example, TCM considers pain, headache and stomachache the result of Qi stagnation.

In TCM theory, blood and Qi are inseparable. Blood is the "mother" of Qi; it carries Qi and also provides nutrients for its movement. In turn, Qi is the "commander" of the blood.

This means that Qi is the force that makes blood flow throughout the body and provides the intelligence that guides it to the places where it needs to be. Blood and Qi also affect one another and have the dynamic ability to transfer various properties back and forth. For example, after labor and delivery, a woman may develop a fever. TCM understands this fever to be related to blood loss, not normally an infection. Losing too much blood causes an overall Qi deficiency. When there is a Qi deficiency, the body cannot function properly and therefore presents with a fever.

Five-Element Theory

TCM believes that the human body is a microcosm of the Universal macrocosm. Therefore, humans must follow the laws of the Universe to achieve harmony and total health. The Yin/Yang and Five-Element theories are actually observations and descriptions of Universal law, not concepts created by man. In ancient times, practitioners of TCM discovered these complex sets of interrelationships that exist on deep energetic levels below the material surface. Over time, these insights developed into a unified body of wisdom and knowledge—TCM theories—and were applied to a way of life and to healing the human body. Even today TCM practitioners use these essential theories to understand, diagnose and treat health problems.

The Five-Element Theory is the bedrock of TCM. It evolved as a way of naming and systematizing patterns of perceived related phenomena, ranging from something as tangible as the weather to more rarified realms such as emotion and capacities of character, into five major groups named for the universal elements: Wood, Fire, Earth, Metal and Water.

The Five-Element Theory states that the five major Organ Systems are:

1. (Liver/Gallbladder,
2. Heart/Small Intestine
3. Spleen/Stomach
4. Lung/Large Intestine
5. Kidney/Urinary Bladder)

Each of the above systems are related to a particular element and therefore to a broad category of correspondences or classifications: from a season of the year to a time of day, to particular colors and foods, etc. Both the Yin/Yang Theory and the Five-Element Theory reflect the entire Universal law in one complete, comprehensive system of related categories.

TCM does not consider the Five Elements themselves to be inert substances. They are fundamental energies alive in nature and always in motion.

The Five-Element Theory encompasses two dynamic relationships—generation and control—that explain how the five major Organ Systems are interconnected. Each element generates, or gives energy to, another. These element pairs are known as mother and child. Each element also restrains or controls another. The proper amount of control keeps all the elements in proportion. With control, one Organ System acts as a feedback loop for its opposite pair as well as its partner organ to keep them functioning smoothly: neither excessively nor deficiently, neither too strongly nor too weakly. These dynamic interactions enable all the Organ Systems to work in one harmonious, greater system. If their relationships are good, a state of wellness prevails; if any of the relationships become unbalanced, health problems result. The Five-Element Theory gives a skilled TCM practitioner a range of options for addressing health problems. For instance, when a patient presents with skin problems, the TCM practitioner understands that the Organ System of the Lung and Large Intestine are involved because the skin is the "tissue" of the Lung, according to the Five Elements.

Therefore, he or she can decide to heal one or both Organs to treat the root cause, not just the symptom of the skin problem.

Meridian Theory

Meridians, or channels, are invisible pathways through which Qi flows that form an energy network that connects all parts of the body, and the body to the universe. TCM understands that our body has twelve major meridians. Each one is related to a specific Organ System.

The meridian network links meridians with each other and connects all body structures—skin, tendons, bone, internal organs, cells, atoms. TCM also understands that meridians connect the interior with exterior and the upper body with the lower body. This interlinked, animating network through which Qi flows freely makes the body an organic whole.

The meridian network is like a system of highways, roads and streets that links major cities. The highways (meridians) and the cities (organs) make up an entire energy map (the body). It is through this system of roadways that energy (Qi) runs.

For example, if a city's internal streets are blocked with traffic, eventually this situation will cause a problem with the highways leading into this city. If the traffic condition worsens, even the cities linked by the major highways will experience a problem. Or, two cities may be fine and traffic may be flowing smoothly within their areas.

Yet, if there is an accident and traffic builds up on one of the roads linking the cities, eventually one or both of these cities will find themselves affected by traffic congestion. This analogy offers a way to understand how blockages in meridians can cause problems in organs.

Meridians form a powerful information system within which each Organ also forms its own data system. In addition to transmitting Qi, meridians also transmit actual information to and among the Organ Systems. It is through the meridians and the flow of Qi that the various parts of the body communicate with each other faster than the speed of light. Interestingly, meridians are also sensitive to time and place.

They reflect and respond to the changing energy of the seasons, the time of day and the climate of a particular place. TCM understands that when the meridian system functions well, the body (including its mind, spirit and emotions) is healthy and maintains homeostasis, a dynamic condition of internal harmony where yin and yang energies operate seamlessly. The ancient medical text Nei Jing states: "The function of the channel (meridian) is to transport the Qi and blood and circulate yin and yang to nourish the body." Because meridians respond to and carry stimulation as well as transmit information, they have the ability to bring healing energy to local, as well as distant, parts of the body. This can create physiological and other changes as Qi circulates. It is this function that makes acupuncture and acupressure work: at specific points along the meridian, the flow of Qi can be enhanced or modified either with needles or with the pressure of the finger or the hands. The energy practice of Qi-gong, with its postures and movements, also affects the flow of Qi.

The energy pathways and the Organ Systems they link provide TCM with a framework for identifying the root cause of health problems and the diagnoses to heal them. Meridians work by regulating the energy functions of the body and keeping it in harmony. If a dysfunction occurs, acupuncture or other therapy can stimulate the relevant meridian(s) to help bring an affected organ back into balance. If Qi stagnates for too long in any meridian, it can become blocked and eventually turn into matter, setting the stage for conditions that can create a physical mass. Dysfunctional meridians can also become susceptible to external pathogenic factors that can migrate to organs along the route of the affected meridian.

TCM Meridian Theory states: "As long as Qi flows freely through the meridians and the organs work in harmony, the body can avoid disease."

Yin / Yang Theory

TCM understands that everything is composed of two complementary energies; one energy is yin and the other is yang. They are never separate; one cannot exist without the other. This is the yin / yang principle of interconnectedness and interdependence; it is not oppositional. The intertwined relationship is reflected in the classic black and white yin / yang symbol.

No matter how you might try to divide this circle in half, the two sections will always contain both energies. The energies themselves are indivisible. From the TCM perspective, this is Universal law at its simplest and deepest.

The Theory of Yin and Yang contains no absolutes. The designation of something as yin or yang is always relative to, or in comparison with, some other thing. For example, the sun and daytime are considered to be yang in relation to the moon and the night, which are yin. However, early morning is yang in comparison to late afternoon, which is more yin. According to the Theory of Yin and Yang, male is yang; female is yin.

Everything in the body is also under the control of the binary system of yin and yang. Because yin and yang have an inseparable relationship, if there is a problem with one, the other will definitely be affected.

Ideally, yin and yang should always remain in harmony, not just in balance. Understanding harmony is an important aspect of understanding TCM. Often, in Western understanding of Complementary and Alternative Medicine (CAM), the term "balance" is described as the desired state, however, in TCM, "harmony" is the ultimate goal.

Although the words "balance" and "harmony" are sometimes used interchangeably, in TCM theory they are quite different: balance is merely the first step toward harmony. Two things can be balanced; they can be of equal proportion or have equal weight, and yet still be separate. Balance has to do with the relationship between two separate entities: for instance, the relationship between the

Heart and Kidney. First, a relationship must be in balance; the next step is to achieve harmony. When two things are in harmony, their energies are not just equally proportioned but blended together into a seamless whole. When two elements exist in harmony, there is an ongoing, unconscious dance between them that happens naturally.

When one predominates, the other recedes; this is homeostasis—internal harmony that is a dynamic condition. In a healthy system, harmony happens naturally —within the body itself, and between the body and external forces of Nature and the Universe. So, when nature's Qi undergoes change as it does seasonally, a person's internal Qi will respond automatically. If, for any reason, it can't make a smooth transition to the energy of the next season, TCM understands that illness will result.

In Western medicine, this lack of harmony can be seen in patients with hot flashes. Those who suffer from this condition during the day have a yang Qi or energy deficiency; those who suffer nightly hot flashes are experiencing a yin Qi deficiency. If a woman experiences hot flashes at both times, then both energies are deficient and must be strengthened.

Many who have had a few bottles of prescription drugs that haven't worked are now trying to find alternatives to modern medicine. If you want to join the growing numbers of people who are working towards alternative medicine, you can look directly into Chinese medicine. There are a variety of practitioners available, all which understand the methods to helping you heal.

If you are familiar with Chinese medicine as an alternative, you may have also noticed that it doesn't seem like there are a lot who are advertising the alternatives. Just because this is true, you don't have to give up hope to finding your options with your health. Through some simple searching, you can find the best way to optimize your health and energy.

The good news about Chinese medicine is that most practitioners that come from the orient are first trained in the ancient practices. Even though it may say that they are specialized in a specific type of practice, you can suspect that they know a few things about the complete picture of Chinese medicine. For example, if you know an acupuncture practitioner, you will be safe in asking about herbal alternatives as well.

Not only can you ask local practitioners about Chinese medicine practices, you can also find other resources that can help. Because alternative medicine is becoming more popular, you can easily find national associations and organizations that are dedicated to promoting alternative methods of Chinese medicine. By linking to these organizations as an alternative, you will be able to expand your possibilities and knowledge of holistic health. Finding a way to link the mind, body and spirit also means finding examples of those who have been initiating alternative health. There are a variety of possibilities that are available, all which can link you to understanding and practicing your flow of energy

Chapter 1:

The Beginnings Of Traditional Chinese Medicine

Alternative medicine and holistic healing are based off of concepts and philosophies of an ancient science. At the root of many holistic practices are the philosophies and ideals that come from Chinese medicine. From the beginnings of this practice has been a growth in natural methods to help promote healing and balance.

The beginnings of Chinese medicine as a practice, come about, in the year 800 BC. Even though the practice began much earlier, it was only recorded beginning at this time through a book known as the "Huang Di Nei Jeng" or "The Yellow Emperor's Classic of Internal Medicine." The methods that were used in this book were based around the herbal remedies that were most significant in helping with holistic healing.

The idea for the "Huang Di Nei Jeng" was based on theYellow Emperor, one of the greatest rulers in Chinese history. He was thought to have lived around 4700 BC, and is often portrayed as a mythical character with the status of royalty that provided inspiration to those living in the orient.

It is through this mythical character that the "Huang Di Nei Jeng" is still portrayed, with the acknowledgement to the Yellow Emperor's knowledge that was passed down holistically.

The beginning of this book included twelve prescriptions through herbs that were used with a combination of twenty-eight different ingredients. By the year 220 BC, the book had become so popular that medical services were established based around the remedies from the Yellow Emperor. The adjustments that were made from this book included detailed classifications of the herbs, how they worked, their strength and what their properties were for healing different ailments.

Overtime, new publications and philosophies were added onto this book in order to provide practitioners with new methods and substances to the basis of the Yellow Emperor's remedy book. These additions provided new insights and books, all the way into the 1700s with the contribution of the Theory of Herbal Medicine.

The ancient practices of Chinese medicine through herbal remedies are a true philosophy that shows how time withstands the ideas of holistic treatments. Through the growth of herbal practices, several in the East have found ways to provide insight and balances between different herbs for better practices to gain energy and balance in one's life.

Chapter 2:

The Five Elements of Oriental Medicine

Similar to the theory of yin-yang, the theory of five elements: wood, fire, earth, metal and water   was an ancient philosophical concept used to explain the composition and phenomena of the physical universe. In traditional Chinese medicine the theory of five elements is used to interpret the relationship between the physiology and pathology of the human body and the natural environment. According to the theory, the five elements are in constant move and change, and the interdependence and mutual restraint of the five elements explain the complex connection between material objects as well as the unity between the human body and the natural world.

In traditional Chinese medicine, the visceral organs, as well as other organs and tissues, have similar properties to the five elements; they interact physiologically and pathologically as the five elements do. Through similarity comparison, different phenomena are attributed to the categories of the five elements

Based on the characteristics, forms, and functions of different phenomena, the complex links between physiology and pathology as well as the interconnection between the human body and the natural world are explained.

The five elements emerged from an observation of the various groups of dynamic processes, functions and characteristics observed in the natural world. The aspects involved in each of the five elements are follows:

Fire: draught, heat, flaring, ascendance, movement, etc.

Wood: germination, extension, softness, harmony, flexibility, etc.

Metal: strength, firmness, killing, cutting, cleaning up, etc.

Earth: growing, changing, nourishing, producing, etc.

Water: moisture, cold, descending, flowing, etc.

One of the major ways in which Chinese medicine determines how one's health is relies on the laws of the universe. This essentially means that any trained person in Chinese medicine will turn towards nature and the characteristics that are in this environment to determine why one may be unhealthy.

One of the ways that these determinations are made is through the five elements.

Between the five elements there exists close relationships that can be classified as mutual promoting and mutual restraining under physiological conditions, and mutual encroaching and mutual violating under pathological conditions. By mutually promoting and restraining, functions of the various systems are coordinated and homeostasis maintained.

By encroaching and violating, pathological changes can be explained and complications predicted.

The order of mutual promoting among the five elements is that wood promotes fire, fire promotes earth, earth promotes metal, metal promotes water, and promotes generates wood. In this way each of the five elements has this type of mutual promoting relationship with the other, thus promoting is circular and endless. According to the order of mutual restraining, however, wood restrains earth, metal restrains wood, etc. Each of the five elements also shares this restraining relationship with the other. Mutual promoting and mutual restraining are two aspects that cannot be separated. If there is no promoting, then there is no birth and growth. If there is no restraining, then there is no change and development for maintaining normal harmonious relations. Thus the movement and change of all things exists through their mutual promoting and restraining relationships. These relationships are the basis of the circulation of natural elements. Encroaching and violating are the pathological conditions of the normal mutual promoting and restraining relationships.

Encroaching denotes that the restraining of one of the five elements to another surpassing the normal level, while violating means that one of the five elements restrains the other opposite to the normal, mutual, restraining order.

The five elements consist of water, wood, fire, earth and metal. When looking at these elements, there are certain attributes that are analyzed. (See page 22) In turn, the analysis that is made will also determine how it is related to various organs. Not only did these five elements determine the relation of the elements to organs, but went on to include things such as how emotions corresponded with these various elements.

The idea behind the five elements is to show how everything is interconnected to each other through the universe. Chinese medicine determines that every man is a reflection of what is in the universe, meaning that each individual can be analyzed in direct co-relation to the elements of the universe.

For Example: if someone is having trouble with their heart or small intestine it would directly relate to Fire. According to Chinese medicine, this would be linked with the qualities of summer and the energy of heat. The result of the heart or intestine trouble would be that the sense organ of the tongue would first be affected. The emotion associated with this would be either joy or shock. The heart and the small intestine will also trigger bitter taste that someone will respond to. The idea is that everything in the external universe is directly aligned with the internal. In order to be completely healthy, or to get holistic health, the five elements principles have to be applied. By doing this, one is able to find the natural solutions for any season or element that they are looking at.

Chapter 3:

Relating the Elements for Holistic Healing

In order for one to be balanced and healthy in Chinese traditions, all of the elements in their body have to be balanced. In order to do this, one must first understand how the elements work together to achieve and maintain complete health. If you are looking towards nature to find a way to heal, then Chinese medicine can help to define what areas you should be looking at.

Not only is the relationship to nature and the body interchangeable, but there are also ways that Chinese medicine uses this relationship in order to help one gain optimal health. By taking the five elements and linking them together, as well as applying them to how one is able to live, there is the ability for one understand how to remain balanced and healthy. After the five elements have been divided and completely understood, they are all put into the proper alignment and place.

This is known as the Shen Cycle, which translates into the Nourishing Cycle. When one is completely balanced and healthy, they can use the cycle of the elements to help.

It is said, according to these Chinese medicine principles that water nourishes wood, wood fuels fire, fire makes earth, and earth yields metal and metal produces water.

Within this same cycle of nourishing, each of the elements can also destroy each other. This is known as Ko, or the Regulating Cycle. When the opposite elements are combined they cancel each other out. Chinese medicine considers both of these cycles to be the natural order of things. They can then take this natural order to help either balance out an imbalanced element in one's body, or help to nourish something that is out of order.

Chinese medicine, at its very roots, carries the philosophy and ideal of combining the natural elements of earth with healing. By cycling together the elements, either through nourishing the elements, or canceling them out, it allows one to keep the natural order in their own life.

It is simply understanding when one's body is in the specific element and understanding how it should respond.

Chapter 4:

Finding Alternative Solutions through the Meridian Systems

One of the most important concepts in Chinese medicine is that every part of the body is linked to another part of the body. Together, these work as an entire system that either functions with a natural flow, or stops in its functioning because it is blocked. If you want to be sure that you are functioning in complete health, you will want to begin to examine the meridian systems.

The meridian systems are used in most Chinese medicine as points that will help to heal. They are most often used in acupuncture and massage that is practiced through professional practitioners of Chinese medicine. These particular points, when measured scientifically, are known to be like pressure points that affect other parts of the human system.

The meridian systems are divided into two categories.

One of these will be on the arms and the other will be on the legs. By pressing these specific points, or massaging them, it affects the internal organs, physical illness, and the flow of energy. The different meridians are also divided into Yin and Yang systems, all that can be affected by positive and negative flows of energy.

The division of the different meridian systems in the arms and legs allows acupuncturists to directly link places in the body that are external with internal organs. For example, an acupuncturist who sees that you have heart trouble will find a Yin meridian on the arm that is directly linked to the heart and treat it in order to begin the flow of energy.

By following the TCM meridian model, one can begin to see the relationship between the internal organs and the external structure of the body. Through the meridian systems, one can determine how the flow of energy needs to be changed and can find ways in which the body is affected through the various organs. This is one of the effective ways to use Chinese medicine for better health.

Chapter 5:

Yoga as Chinese Medicine

There are many different types of yoga, like hatha yoga, karma yoga, bhakti yoga and raja yoga. Yoga techniques use gravity, leverage, and tension through holding poses for varying lengths of time. Ancient texts describe rapid breathing (kapalabhati) as cleansing and stimulating, and slow breathing (nadisuddhi), particularly through alternate nostrils, as calming. Yoga techniques can be learned in classes or through videotape instruction.

On the Western side of the world, Yoga is considered an exercise that helps with strength, cardiovascular and weight loss. However, in Traditional Chinese medicine, Yoga was also used as a practice in order to cultivate health. If you are interested in Yoga, or have begun the practice, you will begin to recognize that Yoga also provides the means for a better balance towards health.

The idea of Chinese medicine is to create a balance of the flow of energy that is happening in one's body. The incorporation of this medicine doesn't just include the balance of the body. It also includes the relationships of the mind and the spirit that relate to the body. All are considered to be intertwined. When the energy flow of one area is off, it changes the energy flow of the entire system. The basis of this idea in Chinese medicine is also the ideal behind Yoga. This form of exercise was used as a method to help with healing and balance in one's life, and can be considered one of the ways to use Chinese medicine.

Yoga is famous for its ability to heal and bring peace of mind. But how does the practice of yoga accomplish this?

There are two nervous systems in the human body: sympathetic and parasympathetic. The sympathetic, commonly known as the "fight or flight" system, causes the blood pressure to rise, the breath rate to quicken, and stress hormones to flood into the body. Historically, this occurred to prepare the body for fighting dangerous animals. But in today's world, we experience this response while we are sitting in traffic or feeling stressed at the office. When this system is overly stimulated, we can experience health consequences such as ulcers, migraines, and heart disease.

The parasympathetic nervous system lowers blood pressure and slows the pace of the breath. When the blood no longer has to rush to the muscles, it is free to travel to the digestive, reproductive, glandular, and immune systems - systems made up of organs that are more necessary to long-term survival. The body now has time to heal the damage accumulated during our daily battles. Studies have shown that long, deep breathing encourages the actions of the parasympathetic nervous system and allows relaxation and healing to occur.

The yogi practices breathing meditations called pranayama, which encourage the actions of the parasympathetic nervous system. So while both the yogi and the cheerleader gain strength and flexibility from practicing backbends and splits, the yogi is able to reap additional health rewards from the addition of pranayama. But even more is happening within the yogi. The yogi is working to calm the fluctuations of the mind.

You probably discovered that your mind wants to think about everything but the breath. Our minds have a tendency to wander, to disconnect from our bodies, to daydream and fret about the future, to reminisce and stew over the past. Humans have evolved the ability to automatically breathe even while sleeping. While breathing does not require conscious awareness, focusing your attention on your breath will force you to focus on what's happening right now, at this very moment. Focusing on your breath doesn't allow your conscious mind to drift away, but encourages it to stay connected in your body and in the now.

But why shouldn't we allow ourselves to daydream or reminisce, it seems harmless? Well, frequently when we are reminiscing about the good old times we begin fear to these events won't occur again. The more time we spend in reverie, the less open we are to the good things that are happening right now. Often, even when we are the midst of a good time, we begin to worry about it ending and start plotting to make it happen again.

We miss out on embracing the moment fully while it is unfolding. And while having goals in life is a good thing, spending hours daydreaming won't get you any closer to making your dreams come true. Being lost in fantasy can often lead to disappointment when reality hits.

The quality of the breath reflects the quality of the mind. There is a connection between our mental, emotional, and psychological states and the pace and depth of our breath. For example, when we are frightened, we take short, quick, shallow breaths. When we are deeply relaxed or asleep, we take long, deep breaths.

While our mental state influences our breathing pattern, we can choose to change our breathing pattern and thereby change our mental state. When you relax and slow the pace of the breath, the pace of the mind is similarly calmed and quieted. Over time, you begin to act and think from a state of peace. The more time you spend in this place, the more likely you are to act with patience, understanding, and compassion.

The breath also helps us to stay connected to the present moment. Staying in the now frees us. We can move on from past grievances and sorrows and can view the world as it really is, without false expectations. We learn to accept ourselves and others as we and they currently are. Being in the moment allows you to be fully present when you spend time with the people you love.

Our mood is also affected by how we feel physically. Ever try to be friendly when you have a stomach ache? Asana helps to keep our muscles, joints, and fascia strong and flexible.

The practice of asana also helps reduce blood pressure, stimulate the immune and glandular systems, reduce insomnia, and heal the body in innumerable other ways.

The simple practices of asana (yoga postures), pranayama (breathing), and drishti (focusing) lead the yoga practitioner to not only a state of optimal physical health, but to a state of peace. These practices help to connect you to the present moment, to others and to your true self.

The practice of Yoga, while it can help to treat ailments, is recognized more often as a way to prevent disease and imbalance. By practicing Yoga, one can keep their health on all levels.

The way that this is done through Yoga is through the opening of the various points in the body with the practice. Every Yoga move is directly linked to various chakras, or points in the body that help with energy flow. Yoga helps to open these chakras, and to help in keeping them open.

By doing so, one is able to increase their energy and begin to stay in better health. Yoga is especially known for helping with problems such as insomnia, and in the functioning of internal organs.

If you want a natural alternative to healing, Yoga as a practice can help. This particular method is known to help increase energy as well as clear blocks that may be in your system. Over time, your energy will begin to increase and flow naturally, allowing you to stay in the best of health without the unnatural twists.

Chapter 6:

Using Science to Prove Chinese Medicine

Even though Chinese medicine has been used as an effective method in China for over 5,000 years, Western scientific proof continues to debate whether this is a logical method to help with healing. If you are interested in Chinese medicine, but are not certain of its effectiveness, you can look at the various research studies that have helped others to reach conclusions about its effectiveness.

The most debated science between East and West is the use of acupuncture as a medicine. At this point in time, the research studies have not led to any complete conclusions about whether acupuncture can be considered a science. At the same time, research indicates that the use of meridians in acupuncture is effective in healing.

Scientists have also stated that because the treatment is harmless, it can be used, and simply needs to have more investigations related to it.

Another debate that has been studied by Western scientists is herbal medicines that are used from traditional Chinese medicine methods. While some of these have not been studied, other parts of the herbs are used in pharmaceutical medications that are prescribed to patients. Chinese wormwood, Ephedra, and artemisinin are some examples of ancient remedies that have moved into Western medicine from Chinese ideals.

Boston University release — Researchers at Boston University School of Medicine (BUSM) and McLean Hospital have found that practicing yoga may elevate brain gamma-aminobutyric (GABA) levels, the brain's primary inhibitory neurotransmitter.

The findings, which appeared in the May issue of the Journal of Alternative and Complementary Medicine, suggest that the practice of yoga be explored as a possible treatment for depression and anxiety, disorders associated with low GABA levels.

The World Health Organization reports that mental illness makes up to 15% of disease in the world. Depression and anxiety disorders both contribute to this burden and are associated with low GABA levels. Currently, these disorders have been successfully treated with pharmaceutical agents designed to increase GABA levels.

What are GABA levels? Gamma-Aminobutyric Acid (GABA) is a neurotransmitter that is inhibitory, that is, it decreases the ability of other neurotransmitters to work. GABA is involved in our level of excitability

Rather than encouraging communication between cells such as Dopamine, Serotonin or Norepinephrine - GABA reduces, discourages, and blocks communication.

This neurotransmitter is important in brain areas involving emotion and anxiety.

When GABA is in the normal range in the brain, we are not overly aroused or anxious. At the same time, we have appropriate reactions to situations in our environment. GABA is the communication speed controller, making sure all brain communications are operating at the right speed

and with the correct intensity. Too little GABA in the brain, the communication becomes out of control, overstimulated, and chemically unstable. Too much GABA and we are overly relaxed and sedated, often to the point that normal reactions are impaired.

American Society of Clinical Oncology release - Two studies report that exercise and yoga can help maintain and in some cases improve quality of life in women with early-stage breast cancer. The first study found that resistance and aerobic exercise improved physical fitness, self-esteem and body composition, and that resistance exercise improved chemotherapy completion rates. The second study demonstrated that yoga was particularly beneficial for women who were not receiving chemotherapy during the study period.

In the first study, Canadian investigators explored the effects of exercise on quality of life, physical fitness and body composition in women receiving chemotherapy for early-stage breast cancer.

This study, the Supervised Trial of Aerobic versus Resistance Training (START) trial, is the largest to date to explore the effects of exercise during chemotherapy and one of the first to evaluate a regimen of resistance exercise. They found that resistance exercise was better than usual care for improving muscle strength, lean body mass and self-esteem.

Aerobic exercise was better than usual care for improving aerobic fitness, self-esteem and body fat percentage. Exercise did not cause lymphedema or other adverse side effects.

In the second study, researchers compared various quality of life measures between 84 women with early-stage breast cancer who took a weekly yoga class for 12 weeks and 44 women who did not take yoga. This was the first study to evaluate the benefits of yoga in an ethnically diverse population of women with breast cancer (primarily Hispanic and African-American women). About half of the women received chemotherapy or radiation therapy during the study period, the remainder had either already completed treatment or not required it. Overall, the women had lower than average levels of quality of life at the beginning of the study.

"Yoga can promote better quality of life for women with breast cancer by helping them connect with others and feel calmer," said lead author Alyson Moadel, PhD, assistant professor in the department of epidemiology and population health at the Albert Einstein College of Medicine. "Because yoga was well-received by all cultural and socioeconomic groups, it has the potential to help many women with early-stage breast cancer."

Among all women in the study, those who did not take yoga reported a drop in social well-being scores (a measure of perceived support from and closeness with others) compared with those who took yoga. All other measures (physical, functional, emotional and spiritual well-being; fatigue; anxiety/sadness; irritability; and confusion) did not differ significantly between the groups. As expected, the benefits of yoga were greater in women who adhered to the prescribed regimen and took more classes.

However, among women not undergoing chemotherapy, those taking yoga reported improved overall quality of life as well as better emotional well-being and mood compared with those not taking yoga, who experienced declines in quality of life, mood, and social and spiritual well-being.

One agreement that all Western research shows, with the various ideas of Chinese medicine, is that the treatments are safe. All of the medical studies indicate that even if the medications are not scientifically proven, they are still not detrimental to one's health and most have few side effects. Because this is a proven point to the holistic methods, most scientists will also state that it is simply a lack of research from the medicine that is used in Chinese philosophies.

From the philosophy to the science, Chinese medication is a debated concept in Western society. However, there is also a growth and a beginning to understanding the concepts that have been used and experimented with over time.

Through the various techniques of Chinese medicine to the continuous use by individuals who are looking for holistic health, Chinese medicine continues to become prominent in Western society.

Let's imagine that you have had a head cold for over a month. No matter what type of medication you try, you simply can't get rid of the problem. It continues to linger, knocking you out of your ability to have the energy you want to and function at the level you want every day. Getting desperate for an answer to get rid of the illness, you begin to look for alternatives.

A friend recommends acupuncture to you in order to help to cure the problem. There happens to be someone that she has also gone to who could probably help you to be cured of your cold. Even though you laugh at first, the cold has dragged on long enough, and you are willing to try the alternatives. You schedule an appointment and get ready to try something a little different.

For most, there is some cynicism on whether the ideas of Chinese medicine really work. Even though it is an ancient practice that has been developed through both the physical and spiritual aspects, it doesn't tie into much science that Western thought would give a second look to.

Chinese medicine, even though it is not a proven science, is a good alternative for those that are dealing with any type of illness. For about 90% that use the method, they will say that there are positive results that come from the practice. All you have to do to see if this is true is to look at the amount of time that it has lasted.

You can also look at the growing popularity of various holistic methods that are now being used. Most of these come from Chinese medical philosophies.

If you are considering an alternative to your health, you can start to turn to ancient philosophies to better your energy. Even though science hasn't proven its validity, time and people have.

Chinese medicine, no matter what level of health you are working towards attaining, can be effective if you walk in with the desire of finding the best healing alternatives.

Chapter 7:

Pathology in Chinese Medicine

A disturbance in the flow of Qi, organ over-or-under activity, and external Qi invading the body are all considered pathological imbalances. They will result in too much or too little Qi (local or systemic) or an erratic flow. Improper flow and amount is the nutshell description of illness in Chinese medicine. But explanations and models of how those two factors come to be are many.

There are three general classes of the causes of illness in Chinese medicine. Internal Pathogenic Qi, External Pathogenic Qi, and Trauma. Internal pathogens are organ dysfunctions, external pathogens are Qi from outside the body which enters the body, and trauma is trauma.

Internal pathogens are the hyperfunction or hypofunction of the internal organs and the emotions. The role of the organs will be more apparent after you read the Functions of Organs: Zang Fu Theory section.

The emotions are the Five Element emotions. Each emotion has a specific affect on the organs of it's element. Anger causes Liver Qi to stagnate. Joy and shock scatter the Heart Qi. Sadness consumes the Lung Qi. Both short and long periods of of emotion can affect the Qi as can intensity of the emotion.

External Pathogen Qi has six types. They're often called the Six Climatic Pathogens because they're named after weather phenomena which possess similar characteristics. The six types are Wind, Heat, Cold, Damp, Dryness, and Summer Heat. Wind is a good example. When Wind enters the body (via the pores in the skin) it attempts to go where it wishes. Invariably this is contrary to the body's healthy flow of Qi and so a struggle arises between the two which impairs or stagnates the Wei Qi.

Trauma damages the main and subsidiary channels causing Qi and Blood to leave the normal currents of flow and accumulate in local tissues.

This accumulation is termed stagnation and the pain which usually accompanies trauma is defined as a consequence of stagnation. If the stagnation's effect is prolonged then other parts of the body which are "downstream" will suffer from the lack of Qi

Wind

You've seen trees in the wind. Wind can appear and disappear very quickly or it can blow steadily. If it's the Lung Qi which is disordered there will be intermittent coughing or paroxysmal coughing. Wind can gradually burgeon in force and speed.

And it moves from place to place. When the Qi is disordered "flu aches" can occur and move from joint to joint. Sometimes a gentle breeze flutters the leaves and sometimes a gale bends the tree over and holds it there. Wind can also cause tremors or paralysis.

Hot & Cold

Hot and Cold are a bit more literal. Both manifest with their actual temperature sensations. They also produce colors in parts of the body; red face, red rashes, red tongue, rusty or red colored urine, and red swellings all indicate the presence of Heat. White, gray or clear indicate the presence of Cold.

Summer Heat

This is a subset of Hot which occurs predominantly during the summer. It's traits are severe heat signs.

Damp

This is moisture. Identifying characteristics are heaviness, thickness, moves downward. Damp excels at blocking Qi.

Dryness

Lack of moisture decreases flexibility in many things. Dryness makes stuff brittle. Paper and bread are two good examples of this. Often bits and pieces of the dry object flake away.

Although these pathogens were identified long before the technology of climate control modern city dwellers are still at risk. Sleeping or working under a vent subjects you to wind. Automobile AC/heat systems set on high create Heat or Cold in extremes to quickly affect a small space. Living in Seattle or south Georgia exposes you to damp and winter in the southwest U.S. subjects you to dryness.

You walk home from work and feel tired. After an eight hour day, your energy can't let you do anything anymore. However, you also know that there are demands to be met as soon as you walk in the door.

If you want to make sure that you can keep up with the activity, you might want to learn how to check your Qi, or energy. If there is a part of your body that is blocked, it can prevent you from getting what you want to done, or having the energy to be alert when you need to be. Starting by finding the flow of your energy, and looking at your pathology, may be able to help.

Pathological imbalances, in Chinese medicine, are known to be a result of your energy being disturbed. This means that your energy is moving too quickly or too slow in your body and in your organs. This is the foundation of Chinese medicine. Changing the flow of your Qi is what will help you to get back to the energy that you want to.

By beginning to understand the relation of pathogens to energy in the body, you can begin to find alternatives to healing. The philosophy basis of Chinese medicine is directly linked to the idea of Qi and how one is able to stay healthy and with energy. If you want to focus your energy on meeting all of your activities, then following the alternatives with Chinese medicine can begin to change your flow in a different direction.

There are a variety of problems that are directly linked to

health in the world today. Everything from mental ailments to physical diseases to problems reflected by other more serious problems are becoming better known. In the increase in knowledge for better health is also the desire to find the correct cures for the problems. Not only are Western scientists trying to find solutions, but traditional Chinese medicine is also working towards increasing the availability of ancient solutions.

Not only is Chinese medicine known to help cure common ailments, but it is now being proven that they are working towards finding alternatives in other ways.

There are several that are turning towards Chinese medicine to help alternate things such as obesity, smoking and addiction to hard drugs.

This is not only a continuation of Chinese medicine, but is also an increase in evidence of the effectiveness of this alternative.

One of the proven effects of Chinese medicine comes from recent research done by a variety of acupuncturists. In this particular study, acupuncture practitioners conducted acupuncture on those who were suffering from obesity and addiction. It was found that there were direct results by refocusing the energy of the person by using specific acupuncture points.

The major change that occurred with the acupuncture is that the chemical of endorphin, which is usually a response to addiction, began to flow differently. This occurred because there were direct pressure points used in the acupuncture that linked to the nervous system. The areas of this nervous system are the ones that carry the endorphins, telling your body that it needs certain things and responds to addictions. Not only are acupuncturists working with those that are addicted in order to open up channels for releasing endorphins into a different direction, but they are also finding ways to use acupuncture in direct areas for the addictions. Ear acupuncture is one of the most well known ways to change the imbalance of endorphins and is done by stimulating specific nerves in the ears, which causes an increase in endorphins and releases the chemical stimulants to stop addictions.

If you are suffering from an addiction, you can try using acupuncture and ancient Chinese medicine in order to help find a cure. Most likely, your body is telling you to release specific chemicals that cause the addiction. By using holistic methods, you can begin to reverse this process and work towards a well-balanced alternative towards your health.

Sometimes, common ailments for not feeling well or functioning at a higher level don't come from the virus that is going around. Most are learning that there is physical pain that is linked to emotional and mental symptoms as well. If you are suffering from a mental pain, and want to find a way to get healing outside of therapy, you can turn to Chinese medicine for help.

Problems with mental health are now being found to directly link to physical pain. One example is with things such as depression. Those who suffer from depression will also commonly have head aches, stomach pains, or have low levels of energy. According to science, as well as Chinese medicine, these mentalities are directly linked to the mind.

There are specific hormones, nerves and chemicals that

are affected by one's mentality. When one is suffering from a specific mental illness, there are different levels of chemicals that are produced to try and rebalance the body. Take the example of depression again. When one is depressed, there will be extra levels of serotonin produced in the mind in order to try to balance this. The effect is that the body becomes imbalanced from the emotion.

Because of the evidence of mental and physical health being linked together, there is also a need to find alternatives for healing. There are several types of medications that are available; however, some find that these simply cause more side effects or don't work. Because of this, there is a turn towards Chinese medicine in order to help cure the problem. By using herbs, massage techniques and even acupuncture, the mental health can begin to change back to a normal level.

If you are suffering from any type of mental imbalance, using holistic approaches may be able to help you find a cure. Chinese medicine will focus directly on finding ways to alternate the flow of energy from the problems and redirect the energy into better mental health. If you are looking for alternatives, Chinese medicine may be a positive cure.

Chinese medicine will always use natural observations in order to determine which parts of the body may be off in their energy. By observing the external functions of the body, they can make assessments on how this affects the internal structure. From here, they will be able to decide on how to change the energy flow.

One of the most important areas of observation for Chinese medicine diagnosis is the pulse.

The different pulses of the body are so important to Chinese medicine, that they are considered an art by learning how to use them appropriately. Usually, only the most trained practitioners can find how to use the pulse properly.

The reason why the pulse is important to the observations is because Chinese medicine has found connections between the pulse and every area of the body. In Western medicine, there is an understanding that the pulse of the heart is located in the wrist and also the neck.

In Chinese medicine, there are also pulses for the kidney, liver, and other body areas.

Not only do all of the internal organs have specific pulses in different areas of the body, but these also have different depths. This means that a reading of a pulse can be heard in 'layers' in each position. Typically, each pulse will have three different depths that can be observed. These can be found in nine different areas when the diagnosis is being made from pulse.

If a practitioner is looking for a diagnosis for a pulse, they will look for several attributes. If you are in Chinese medicine, you will most likely know about twenty-eight different characteristics to look for. These may be related to how the pulse sounds, the rate it is beating at, and other factors such as this.

The characteristics that are determined will also help to draw conclusions about which areas of the body are off of their regular energy flow.

If you are moving into Chinese medicine, expect your

pulse to be checked. This is one of the main considerations in Chinese medicine, and is never over looked in the diagnosis. The art of checking the pulse in Chinese medicine is one of the main foundations for understanding how the internal Qi of someone is functioning.

Because Chinese medicine is a method that doesn't use technology, check the heart rate and hook you up to a monitor, it is hard to see how a practitioner can find what you need. If you are looking into Chinese methods as an alternative, you may also want to find how a practitioner can determine where your Qi is off and what type of help you need.

You can use basic tools for your own diagnosis as well if you are trying to find a remedy to give you more energy and more well-being. The basic principle that will be used when determining a diagnosis for your health is to find physical affects that are causing differences in how you function.

The rule of thumb for anyone practicing Chinese medicine is that the exterior is guidance to what is happening in the interior. Most practitioners will use what they see as a way to speak with what your body needs.

Because Chinese medicine will use the exterior as a basis, you will most likely be taken through a series of questions that help to determine your condition. These questions are based on a series of ten categories, and can consist to up to one-hundred questions.

All of these will reflect parts of the Qi that need to be worked on. The categories of these questions are temperature, perspiration, digestion, sleep energy, exercise, urine, thirst, appetite, reproduction and stools.

From here, practitioners will look at various areas of your body to see how they are not working or working together. To begin, a diagnosis will be made on how you are breathing. This includes both the steadiness of your breath and the way that your voice sounds. The smell of your body will also be diagnosed in order to make sure that your temperature elements are balanced.

After this, you will have various other areas of your body looked at to see how they are balanced or imbalanced. Diagrams for the tongue are important as they are seen as a reflection of the way in which the internal system is working. Practitioners will also listen to your pulse to see what the rate is and to see if it is even in comparison to the rest of your body functions.

By examining the various parts of your body, a practitioner is able to find what is best for you and what parts of your body are either imbalanced or not receiving the right amount of energy.

From this point, they are able to use the proper methods in moving things back to a normal pace. The proper diagnosis in Chinese medicine is working from the outside in.

Traditional Chinese medicine is the idea that everything is interconnected in one's body and in the universe. Through this concept, there was a development of the way in which the system could be divided.

The understanding of this system is what allowed one to practice alternatives towards health and balanced energy.

The Zang-Fu theory is the concept that the functions of the different organs interact with each other. This interaction allows them to function in different ways, and also balances out the health of different individuals. When one's internal organs are completely balanced, they have reached complete health because their energy is able to flow naturally and without any blocks.

From this major concept, the internal organs are divided into various categories. The first set of categories is the Zang, which are the Yin organs. This includes the heart, liver, spleen, lungs, kidneys, and pericardium. The Fu are the Yang organs and includes the intestines, gall bladder, urinary bladder and stomach. Each of these organs will be paired together; meaning that one Yang organ corresponds to one Yin organ.

Through each of these categorizations, the organs are able to correspond and function by relating to each other. When these organs are not functioning properly together, it will be the cause of dysfunction in the body. Beyond this, it is the functioning of these organs that directly link to the way that the mind and the spirit function together. The Zang organs will be directly linked with specific emotions as well as senses. The Fu system is the opposite of this because it is linked to the hollow system and digestion.

The combination of all of the elements of the body is the major concept in the Zang Fu theory. By combining the internal organs and discovering the relationships that they have between each other, one is able to find the necessary answers to healing. Chinese medicine, through combining all of the elements is able to work towards an internal healing that leads to external functions of health.

The idea of connectedness between the universe and the system of a human is at the basis of philosophies for Chinese medicine. If you have ever heard of the basics for any type of Oriental practice, you are also familiar with the idea of the connection between the physical, mental and spiritual ideas.

If you want to learn how these can work together holistically and for your health, you don't have to look any further than Chinese medicine.

The idea of connecting all of the elements in your body for optimum health is known as Shen. This comes from the idea that all of the elements in the universe are interconnected and related to one's body. When taking the ideas of the elements of the universe and incorporating them into how a human is interconnected.

The first point of focus in order to connect Shen is the one that is related to waking consciousness. According to the Shen philosophy, this consciousness is in the heart. Everything that is related to heart health, under this method, is also linked with the consciousness needing to wake up.

The next part of Shen is the spirit. According to this science, the spirit is located in the liver. In Chinese, this is referred to as the Ethereal Spirit. The next Shen is the soul of the body, also known as the corporeal soul. This resides in the lungs of one's body. Intellect, or Yi is in the spleen and Will, meaning the urge to do something is in the kidney. The idea of this particular system is to combine the elements of the physical with the elements of the mind and the spirit. By doing this, one is able to find the physical elements and work on two approaches to healing a person through physical and spiritual at the same time. Combining the mind, spirit and body together is the basis of all Chinese medicine and philosophy. By learning to combine these, one is able to find the best approaches to healing a person in a holistic method. Using Shen, the concept of elements of the universe, and seeing how they relate as a system to the body, allows one to find a way to become unified within themselves.

The holistic approach to medicine doesn't just include sticking needles in your body or taking an extra set of herbs every day.

It also consists of finding an approach to your life that will lead to a well rounded well being.

If you are working towards healing, gaining energy or just feeling better about your every day life, than approaching Chinese medication is a great way to begin approaching your life differently.

Along with the diagnosis and assessments of your physical body, is the connection to the mind and spirit within Chinese medicine. Because this is an important concept in Chinese medication, meditation will often be used as a basis for many of the practices. This is especially seen in practices such as Qi-gong and Yoga, where meditation combines with physical movement in order to open the energy centers of the body.

If you are working towards achieving balance in your physical life, then you will want to begin by opening the body centers through meditation. Even though this is often considered a mental and spiritual practice, it will also affect you physically. The idea of breath in any Chinese medicine is important, as it clears several of your centers. This is one of the elements that are never ignored in Chinese medicine. Not only will your breath begin to clear your body centers, but it is also proven that the meditation methods will help to improve other areas of your body. Scientific research has begun to study meditation and how its applications can directly affect your well being. When you breathe deeply, the extra oxygen will cleanse your system and will also move into areas of your body that need the extra oxygen. It will also begin to affect your nervous system by stimulating chemicals in your body. Over time, the meditation practices can detoxify your entire system, helping you to be more energized in your daily life.

If you are looking into the practices of Chinese medicine, you will also want to consider meditation. This practice can't be separated from Chinese medicine or holistic health.

By approaching the mental and spiritual aspects of the medicine, as well as the physical, you will be able to enjoy a well-rounded approach towards the ancient medical practice.

If your body is out of sync with what it is supposed to be doing, it can cause endless problems. You may feel tired all of the time, or restless. For no apparent reason, you may get headaches or feel nauseous during the day. Beyond this, you can catch the viruses and colds going around all of the time.

According to Chinese medicine, this simply means that your flow of energy is off. If this is the case, and you want to find an alternative method to getting back in touch with what your body needs, you don't have to look any further than Chinese medicine. One of the methods that can be used for Chinese medicine is Tuina, also known as Oriental bodywork therapy. Tuina originated around 1700 BC in order to help with children's diseases that were directly related to the muscles and skeletal system of children. The concept of Tuina was also developed for help with digestion for adults. After the year 600, the concept of Tuina was considered to be an art, and was banished by the government. It wasn't until the beginning of the Communist regime in the 1960s that it became popular again as a method for medical arts.

Tuina is like a combination of acupuncture and massage. (Tuina is being included here only for that reason.) A practitioner will work on changing the flow of your energy in your body by using various hand techniques. The hand techniques will first be used in order to massage the tissues and muscles of your body. Afterward, specific points, also used for acupuncture will be focused on. This added pressure is known to change the flow of Qi. After this, the practitioner will focus on realignment of the bones, skeletal structure and ligaments in order to realign them.

Beyond these basic techniques, practitioners may also choose to combine herbs, salves and ointments to enhance the Tuina. This will help to completely shift all levels of the energy systems that are in your body, allowing you to become more generated, balanced and healthy.

If you are looking for an alternative method to get to the depths of your health, Tuina is the method you will want to look into. This particular method is known to heal those that use it on all levels, with a combination of Chinese medicine techniques that are popular. By doing this, there is the ability for those using it to change their energy flow into better health.

The growth in medicine and technology has also made significant growth in possibilities to stay in good health. There are medications for sleeping and staying awake, relaxing and gaining energy, headaches and an imbalance of systems. All of these medications begin to pump various things into your system that your body then is forced to react to, sometimes not so naturally.

If you want to take a different approach to your healing, why not try a more natural remedy? Chinese medicine understands how the body can be naturally healed, and has developed a variety of methods to help bring this into place. One of the popular methods used are traditional healing massages. Not only will this help you to heal by clearing up blocks that may be making you ill, but it will also help you to relax in the process.

The Chinese traditional healing massage was developed over 2500 years ago in the orient. Through this development was an understanding of how the human touch, combined with specific pressure points could help to stop disorders.

Each of these touches would stimulate specific areas of the body that were not in tune with the natural flow of energy. This would then allow one to begin there own healing process.

Not only did massages begin to develop various reactions to touch, but they also began to develop into focus points for healing. For example, many of the traditional massages for healing will be focused on the abdominal area in order to help balance out internal organs. Other parts of the massage will focus on the tissues and muscles that may not be receiving the proper nutrients or flow of energy.

The idea of Chinese medicine is one that moves beyond the prescription pills and into a method of complete relaxation. By doing this, one is able to find an alternative method to begin healing and developing a holistic approach to health. The various massages that have been developed through Chinese medicine are a great way for you to stop taking the extra medications, and instead, sit back and relax.

If you have ever heard of ideas from physical fitness or Yoga, then you are familiar with the idea of using the energy in your body properly. In Chinese Medicine, the energy that you have is something that is much deeper than a physical fitness. The idea if Qi (Chi) is an energy force that is often referred to in order to stay healthy.

The idea of Qi begins with elements that are in the use universe that make up energy. This same Qi that is in the universe is, by Chinese medicine philosophy, also in ever living being. The Qi that is being referred to is something that Chinese philosophy considers to be in every part of every thing. It can't be destroyed, only changed.

One way to explain the way that Qi functions in Chinese philosophy is through the element of water. Under certain conditions, water will change into ice or evaporate. Even though it is changing form or place, it still functions as the same type of energy in the other form.

Through the idea of energy being in everyone's being, and changing as the person needs, is the relation to how this can be used for medicine. All of the Qi that is moving through the body has currents that the energy flows through, much like the circulation system. The Chinese medicine system states that there are fourteen major points where the Qi flows through a person. All of these points will have Yin and Yang access to them and are used in practices such as acupuncture. As the system of Qi flows through someone, it also functions within the body to specific areas. When all of your Qi is flowing properly then you are considered healthy. Not only does your Qi track your energy, it also makes sure that the different systems that are functioning transform the different parts of the body so they are balanced. For example, some types of Qi will take nutrients to the muscles. It is also known to keep parts of the body protected from the wrong types of food, while other areas of the body contain the elements that are needed.

The idea of Qi is to keep the energy of the body functioning in the proper way. When one is in complete health, they are known to have reached Upright Qi. By keeping everything flowing in the right manner, and paying attention to how the body is changing, there will be the ability to continue to hold the energy of the universe in one's body.

Chapter 8:

The Practice of Qigong as Chinese Medicine

The use of meditation as a form of healing is one of the most important concepts used in Chinese medicine. From ancient practices, it is believed that meditation links one to their energy, allowing them to remain clear thinking and have a better energy flow.

Qigong is one of the most popular medical meditation practices used for Chinese medicine. From its origins, it has been known to be not only a meditation, but also a self-medicating practice by moving the flow of energy, or Qi.

QiGong refers to a wide variety of traditional "cultivation" practices that involve methods of accumulating, circulating, and working with chi or energy within the body. Qigong is sometimes mistakenly said to always involve movement and/or regulated breathing; in fact, use of special methods of focusing on particular energy centers in and around the body are common in the 'higher level' or evolved forms of Qigong. Qigong is practiced for health maintenance purposes, as a therapeutic intervention, as a medical profession, a spiritual path and/ or component of Chinese martial arts.

The 'Qi' in 'Qigong' means breath or air in Chinese, and, by extension, 'life force', 'dynamic energy' or even 'cosmic breath'. 'Gong' means work applied to a discipline or the resultant level of skill, so 'Qigong' is thus 'breath work' or 'energy work'. Attitudes toward the scientific basis for Qigong vary markedly. Most Western medical practitioners and many practitioners of traditional Chinese medicine, as well as the Chinese government, view Qigong as a set of breathing and movement exercises, with possible benefits to health through stress reduction and exercise. Others see Qigong in more metaphysical terms, claiming that cosmic Qi can be drawn into the body and circulated through channels (meridians).

The energy flow of Qi is that which enables one to have the energy that they need on all levels, leading to a practice of Qigong, which helps one to focus their energy on what is needed.

When one practices Qigong, they focus on specific focal points of the body. This allows the practitioner to clear these points and continue to stay balanced, energized and healthy.

Qigong is best known for combining within itself, the ideas of meditation, breathing and movement. This begins with a series of breathing exercises that are used in order to begin the flow of energy. This is then combined with exercises that allow the muscles to become tense and relax. These exercises are known to help the muscles to become heated, which in turn, allows for an increase in producing energy and digesting nutrients that are needed throughout the body.

When one is beginning Qigong, there will be a focus on deep breathing as well as meditation of visualizations and clearing of the mind. This purpose is to begin creating a discipline in the rhythms in one's body. The idea is that this will then begin to reflect the rhythms of life that is surrounding a person. The result will be an elimination of tension of nerves, irregularities and dysfunctions in the body. The long term result of this will be strengthening and balance of the body. The main purpose behind Qigong is to activate channels of energy that are in every person. This is a holistic healing technique that everyone has the ability to practice, either as a meditation or a way to develop a strengthening of the entire system. The combination of meditation techniques with movement allows one to become in sync with the rhythm of their own body and life, giving them a holistic and balanced way of living.

Chapter 9:

Chinese Food Therapy

" If we eat wrongly, No doctor can cure us; if we eat
rightly, No doctor is needed."

- Victor G. Rocine circa 1930

Food Therapy has a recorded history of more than 3,000
years and is the most basic treatment in Chinese Medicine
to prevent and cure disease. It is the preparation of
medicinal food dishes, using selected food ingredients and
superior herbs, to derive the necessary nutrients to treat
specific health conditions. It is the product of accumulated
experience from generation after generation of close
monitoring and refinement of recipes on people. Each recipe
is tried-and-true and the natures, characteristics,
therapeutic effects and impacts on people are fully known.
Besides, most recipes are very delicious and they are
specialties in the Chinese cuisine.

There are hundreds of these recipes in circulation and many households are using them on a regular basis. The recipes can be classified into the following categories:

1. Health promotion to improve health on a regular basis.
2. Sickness prevention to prevent seasonal climate related problems.
3. Disease control to fight early symptoms of health problems.
4. Supporting to complement the primary treatment and to combat adverse side effects of harsh drugs during sickness.
5. Recuperating to revive and regain vitality after sickness.
6. Rejuvenating to repair damages and body malfunctions to restore health.

Eating foods with medicinal effects to meet our health conditions is the most effective way in promoting good health. If you are on a quest for good health, we strongly recommend that you include medicinal foods in your diet. They are less expensive than drugs, have no adverse side effects, are easy to make, and are extremely nutritious and tasty. They also make your meals more interesting. The benefits are no other foods or drugs can match.

You are what you eat! If you take charge of your health by eating knowledgeably, you can have a healthy life. Your immune system can protect you from infectious disease. You can delay the onset of degenerative disease and defy aging. Nourish your body well and it will serve you well much longer.

Chinese food therapy dates back as early as 2000 BC.

However, proper documentation was only found around 500 BC.

The Yellow Emperor's Classic of Internal Medicine also known as the Niejing, which was written around 300 BC, was most important in forming the basis of Chinese food therapy.

It classified food by four food groups, five tastes and by their natures and characteristics.

During the Chau dynasty (16 BC), food therapy was established as a specialist field. The state even had a food specialist serving the emperor in the imperial court. It was during the Tang dynasty (608-906 AD) that food therapy became popular and the classic books on the subject were published.

Throughout Chinese history, healthcare was not the responsibility of the state but rather the responsibility of every ordinary citizen. People used their own resources to find cures when they became sick, which meant that most people could not afford to be sick. This is why preventive healthcare is so popular in China. Out of the four pillars of health lifestyle, diet, exercise and mind , diet is the most important because food is considered the primary cause of sickness as well as the main reason for living long and healthy.

Food plays a center role in Chinese culture. Cooking good food for family members is a lifelong profession for most women. Children are brought up with some knowledge of the nature of their daily foods. Dietary restriction is commonly understood and observed. Eating well and healthy is almost a national obsession and definitely the most valued activity of family life.

communicating to you how to use your food and balance it out properly. If your body is unbalanced, you can use food to recreate a proper balance. For example, some foods may cause your energy to be lower. You can use roots of foods in order to increase this, which are directly linked to the Yang foods.

Ginseng is one popular example that will help to increase circulation and the metabolism. This is one of several examples that can help you to heal and balance naturally.

Next time you are ready to eat your meal, make sure that you have both Yin and Yang in combination with each other. Over time, you will notice that the balance of your energy, as well as the various effects of the food makes a difference in how you function. Using Chinese food therapy as a method of health is one of the easiest ways to help chewing in your health.

Using herbs to fight against diseases is an old custom going back thousands of years in China. Ancient Chinese herbalists tested herbs for safety and efficacy on themselves instead of on animals. From generation to generation, our pioneers sought for the knowledge and experiences about herbs and diseases at the risk of losing their own lives in this great enterprise for people's health. Based on this priceless knowledge and the experiences accumulated for thousands of years an experimental medical science called Traditional Chinese Medicine (TCM). In terms of Traditional Chinese Medicine there are many balances not only between human and the natural world, but also inside our body. Problems come when the balances are broken. Chinese herbs could be used in combination to adjust entirely and systematically all these different balances.

You go into your kitchen after a long day's work and open the refrigerator. The availability of food isn't looking good for you again. It's either left over pizza, or another microwave meal. You find the fastest and easiest solution so that you can continue with your day and not let the food stop you from getting what you need to done.

According to Chinese medicine, this can be one of the major causes of illness. Not eating balanced and properly can lead to a stop in the right energy flow in your body, causing your body to not have the ability to process its nutritional needs correctly. The alternative that is suggested is Chinese food therapy, where there is a balance between the food that you eat and the nutrition that you get.

The philosophy behind Chinese food therapy is that everything must be balanced. This begins by discovering the polar opposites of foods that are available and combining them for a middle ground. Yin and yang are the philosophy that is used for foods, giving the best combination of elements for health. Yang is known to increase body heat, which will raise the metabolism to process nutrients.

Yin then combines with this to decrease the body heat, which will balance the nutrients that are being processed in the metabolism.

In order for Chinese food therapy to work properly, there has to be an understanding of how your body reacts to specific things. If you are completely balanced, too much of either yin or yang will cause a reaction in your body, allowing you to stay balanced. Everything that your body does, when using Chinese food therapy, will be

In this way Chinese herbs could be used for different symptoms caused by different factors at the same time without affecting the normal function of our body.

The most powerful feature of Traditional Chinese Medicine is that it allows you to easily combine multiple ingredients to form a recipe to suit the specific need of individual. Chinese herbs should not be used in form of standard industrial products manufactured in bulk to cope with all body issues. Only custom-made is the traditional and professional way to use Chinese herbs to address the individual symptoms exactly.

TCM always focused on the obvious symptoms much more than on the elusive pathology. By watching and inspecting the abnormal changes of our common conditions, such as breath, pulse, energy, sleep, sweat, appetite, urine, stool, influence by and response to heat/ cold/ wet/ dry, tongue and tongue coating color, etc., Chinese herbs could be easily used for effecting diseases even though the causes and mechanisms of the disease were still unknown. This great feature puts TCM in an advantageous position in fighting against refractory diseases which people have little knowledge of.

In Chinese medicine everything has a place and a structure in order to help with healing. All of these are natural approaches to bringing holistic health in an individual. One of the concepts that Chinese medicine uses in relation to this is herbal remedies. By combining a variety of elements, there is the ability for the herbs to help in healing everything.

The basis behind herbal remedies is to combine a series of herbs in order to bring about the desired effect. Usually, there will be a formula of four herbs used in combination with each other. This is done in order to treat secondary illnesses that may have been affected by the primary illness. It also helps to balance and strengthen the body while it is healing.

When Chinese medicine begins to divide the various herbal remedies, they will do so by a hierarchy. At the top of this hierarchy is the emperor herb. This will be used to cure the major illness that is taking place. Underneath this is the 'ministers' of the herbal remedy. This is used to treat any secondary illnesses that are taking place. After this, herbal 'assistants' will be used to support the other two herbs. The last set of herbs will be the messenger herbs, which will tell the primary and secondary herbs where to go and how much of an effect to take on the body.

The herbal remedies that are placed together after this will be divided by the specific symptoms that are being seen. Like all other parts of Chinese medicine, these will first be found through the five elements and how they relate to the body. For example, some herbs will be spicy in order to relate to areas of the body that need this extra element to begin better flow of Qi.

The last part of herbal medicine from ancient Chinese remedies is to determine the type of energy that is needed by a person. This is found by diagnosis and examining the Qi that is in a person. After this, a specific mixture of these four hierarchies will be mixed together in order to help change the energy flow that is in someone. By examining the Qi and finding respective remedies through herbs, one is able to find the best solutions using a holistic method. This allows one to benefit from the use of Chinese medicine and herbs in order to fight off an illness.

Chapter 10:

Acupuncture and Chinese Medicine

If you are like most, you may not see the pleasure in being treated with needles poking into your skin. However, to those in Chinese medicine, and to several who have discovered alternatives with holistic healing, this is the perfect remedy. The idea of acupuncture in Chinese medicine is important to help with healing the energy flow in someone.

Acupuncture is based on the idea that there are certain points in the body that can help one to heal. When these points in the body receive extra pressure through a device, they will be able to assist with the healing.

In the practice of Acupuncture, needles will be used as the major transports to reconnect the energy flow in the body. The use of acupuncture begins by studying the various areas that the flows of energy are located in. These are known as meridians or channels in the body. The body has twelve major meridans where energy will flow and cycle. The places where these channels connect are usually where energy can become blocked off. By using acupuncture, the connecting areas for the channels are examined and unblocked by pressuring the specific points.

Once one has found the connections for the acupuncture, then it is important to find the effects that all of these connections have. Each different point will have elements that are linked directly to what the body needs in order to stay balanced. These are specifically linked to the five elements that are considered to be the basis for the laws of the universe.

By finding the various channels and connections in the body, acupuncture specialists are able to find which areas of Qi are not flowing properly. This allows them to effect the way that the body flows in order to help restore and revitalize the energy levels in the body. By getting one into a better flow of their energy, they can achieve complete health.

Usually, science driven societies are optimistic about the ideas linked to acupuncture and their effectiveness. Even though this ancient practice has become more known in the past ten years, it is still a procedure that is not completely understood. By understanding how the process is done, the possible side effects and the outcome, you can determine if this ancient Chinese medicine practice is right for you. The experience of getting acupuncture done, despite what many think, is not as painful as it looks. Acupuncture is generally painless when you are going through the process. Usually, the effects will be no more noticeable than a mosquito bite, but this is even considered rare.

Most likely, going through the process of acupuncture will either give you more energy or cause you to relax into a state of meditation.

During the procedure, you can expect the acupuncturist to be prepared with several practical things. The needles that are used will generally be of an inch to several inches long.

The needles are made out of sterilized silver, stainless steel or copper and are considered safe by the same standards used in any hospital.

In order to ensure that the needles are safe, there are several places that will regulate what is being used. The National Commission for the Certification of Acupuncture and Oriental Medicine has a specific department that ensures that all needles that are used are sterile and safe. If you want to be certain, you can make sure that the person you go to has a CNT, also known as a Clean Needle Technique Certification. This will ensure that there are no problems with the procedure in terms of other health issues.

Of course, there are still other risks that may occur. By standards of other procedures, acupuncture is not as risky. The most serious problem may be a punctured organ. However, these are uncommon with most practices. This is the only major problem that one may run into. Beyond this, the only possibilities for problems may be things such as dizziness, nausea or bruising.

If you are considering acupuncture as an option for any possible reason, you will also want to make sure you know exactly what you are getting into. Overall, acupuncture is considered to be a safe process, as well as helpful in relieving any kind of imbalance or misguided energy. Before walking into this ancient Chinese medicine practice, you will want to make sure that you know the procedure and the possible outcomes. Acupuncture is an ancient Chinese technique that is used to help restore health. By focusing on specific points in the body, acupuncturists are able to find the way in which the body's energy is flowing and find new ways to make sure that everything flows properly. This helps one to remain balanced and holistically healthy.

Most of us know that acupuncture will find specific points in the body and place needles in that area in order to restore or unblock energy in the body. Understanding the different points that an acupuncturist looks for will help one to understand why the different points of the body and how these link together in this form of Chinese medicine.

The first set of points that are used in acupuncture are transporting points. There are five known transporting points that are focused on throughout the body. These will mostly be found in the legs and arms. Each of these transporting points is named after characteristics of water, and all hold the same characteristics that a water form would. For example, the sea is where the points connect energy with the body to the organs because it is a set of deeper points in the body.

From here, the points will be determined by the five elements of the earth. These are usually found at finger and toe tips in the body. For an acupuncturist, it is important that the five elements are represented and flowing with the right Qi in all of the points that they should be found.

If you have ever seen acupuncture at work, you know that the needles will all be placed into a person's body at different lengths. This also links directly to the points that are being examined in the body.

The shallowest set of points is known as the Xi-Accumulating Cleft Points. These are wider and shallower spots that make it easy for Qi to become blocked. The upper third of the body has a special set of points that will be used.

These are known as the window to sky points and are directly linked to one's spirit and relationship from heaven to earth.

Mu-Front-Alarm Points are also examined. These are in the front of the body and are also associated with organs. Only the organs that have been diagnosed as blocked will have needles placed to help their flow. Of course, everything that is done to the front also has to be done to the back. Shu-Back Points are the points that correspond with the front diagnosis, only on the other side of the body.

Knowing the different points as an acupuncturist is one of the most important parts of understanding how to heal. By beginning this process and finding the points that need different types of Qi unblocked, one will begin to feel the difference and begin to heal.

Acupuncture is the most common type of healing that is done with the help of someone who is trained in the healing methods. There are also herbal medicine remedies that are used along with moxibustion. Moxibustion is the burning of herbs, instead of using them as a remedy, and is often associated with aromatherapy.

Cupping, which is close to the practice of acupuncture or massage is also a common method that is done in order to get your Qi moving in the right direction again.

No matter what type of healing remedy you feel that you need, Chinese medicine can find an alternative and holistic approach to helping. If you are working towards better energy levels, feel ill or are looking for a new method to going to the doctor, than finding the right type of Chinese medicine as a method is an easy place to start without the side effects.

Chapter 11:

The Principle of Yin and Yang in Chinese Medicine

Chinese medicine is not only a way of science that incorporates the discoveries made in holistic health. It also incorporates philosophies that are important for one to be able to stay in the best health. Along with these philosophies are practical principles that are applied with Chinese medicine in order for holistic health to be achieved.

In Chinese medicine, health is represented as a balance of yin and yang. These two forces represent the bipolar manifestation of all things in nature, and because of this, one must be present to allow the other to exist. Hence, where there is above there is below, whatever has a front also has a back, night is followed by day, etc. On an emotional level, one would not know joy had they never experienced pain. It is important to note that the balance of yin and yang is not always exact, even when the body is healthy. Under normal circumstances the balance is in a state of constant change, based on both the external and internal environment. For example, during times of anger, a person's mood is more fiery, or yang, and yet once the anger has subsided, and a quiet peaceful state is achieved, yin may dominate.

This shift in the balance of yin and yang is very natural. It is when the balance is consistently altered, and one (be it yin or yang) regularly dominates the other, that health is compromised, resulting in illness and disease.

Traditional Chinese medicine practitioners attempt to determine the exact nature of the imbalance, and then correct it through the use of acupuncture, herbal remedies, exercise, diet and lifestyle. As balance is restored in the body, so is health.

The philosophical origins of Chinese medicine have grown out of the tenets of Daoism (also known as Taoism). Daoism bases much of its thinking on observing the natural world and the manner in which it operates, so it is no surprise to find that the Traditional Chinese medical system draws extensively on natural metaphors. In Chinese medicine, the metaphoric views of the human body based on observations of nature are fully articulated in *The Theory of Yin-Yang* and the *System of Five Elements.*

The direct meanings of yin and yang in Chinese are bright and dark sides of an object. Chinese philosophy uses yin and yang to represent a wider range of opposite properties in the universe: cold and hot, slow and fast, still and moving, masculine and feminine, lower and upper, etc. In general, anything that is moving, ascending, bright, progressing, hyperactive, including functional disease of the body, pertains to yang.

The characteristics of stillness, descending, darkness, degeneration, hypo-activity, including organic disease, pertain to yin.

The function of yin and yang is guided by the law of unity of the opposites. In other words, yin and yang are in conflict but at the same time mutually dependent. The nature of yin and yang is relative, with neither being able to exist in isolation. Without "cold" there would be no "hot"; without "moving" there would be no "still"; without "dark", there would be no "light". The best example of yin-yang interdependence is the interrelationship between substance and function. Only with ample substance can the human body function in a healthy way; and only when the functional processes are in good condition, can the essential substances be appropriately refreshed.

The idea of Yin and Yang is one of the many principles that are at the root of Chinese medicine and it's functioning. This particular method was applied through Taoism, one of the religious practices in the Orient. From this philosophy, the Chinese discovered that the laws of the universe could be applied to each individual in order to gain optimum health.

The opposites in all objects and phenomena are in constant motion and change: The gain, growth and advance of the one mean the loss, decline and retreat of the other. For example, day is yang and night is yin, but morning is understood as being yang within yang, afternoon is yin within yang, evening before midnight is yin within yin and the time after midnight is yang within yin. The seed (Yin) grows into the plan (Yang), which itself dies back to the earth (Yin). This takes place within the changes of the seasons.

Winter (Yin) transforms through the Spring into Summer (Yang), which in turn transforms through Autumn into Winter again. Because natural phenomena are balanced in the constant flux of alternating yin and yang, the change and transformation of yin-yang has been taken as a universal law.

Traditional Chinese medicine holds that human life is a physiological process in constant motion and change. Under normal conditions, the waxing and waning of yin and yang are kept within certain bounds, reflecting a dynamic equilibrium of the physiological processes. When the balance is broken, disease occurs. Typical cases of disease-related imbalance include excess of yin, excess of yang, deficiency of yin, and deficiency of yang.

The idea of Yin and Yang incorporates five major ideas that are then used in order to help one gain the best of health. The first of these is opposition. This means that everything and everyone has two polar opposites.

When one is balanced, both of these are controlling each other. This opposition is essential to one being able to exist in the universe. Not only is this opposition essential for existence, but it is also what allows one to be healthy. By balancing out these two opposites, one is able to nourish them as well as grow into new understanding and balance. However, even if these are not balanced, there is still a little of one side into the other making the idea of Yin and Yang interchangeable.

When one applies these particular philosophies to health, they can find that they are able to use the principles to help with health. With each side of your body is another side that is the polar opposite.

A good example is your abdomen, which needs your back in order to remain balanced. By focusing on both sides, you will be able to gain balance, energy and a holistic approach to your life.

The idea of Chinese medicine is one that doesn't just record symptoms through a scientific perspective. It takes into account the dark and light sides of everyone. By learning how to apply the principles of Yin and Yang to every part of your health, there is the ability to learn to exist with a new balance.

For Further Reading

1. Voices of Qi: An Introductory Guide to Traditional Chinese Medicine by Alex Holland and Fred Lanphear (Paperback - Jan 27, 2000)

2. The Web That Has No Weaver : Understanding Chinese Medicine by Ted J. Kaptchuk (Paperback April 11, 2000)

3. Traditional Chinese Medicine: An Authoritative and Comprehensive Guide by Henry C. Lu (Paperback   Jul 20, 2005)

4. The Foundations of Chinese Medicine: A Comprehensive Text for Acupuncturists and Herbalists. Second Edition by Giovanni Maciocia (Hardcover - Jul 13, 2005)

5. Practical Diagnosis in Traditional Chinese Medicine by Tietao (Hardcover - Jun 11, 1999)

6. Fundamentals of Chinese Medicine: Zhong Yi Xue Ji Chu (Paradigm Title) by Nigel Wisemann and Andy Ellis (Paperback - Sep 1995)

7. Complete Illustrated Guide to Chinese Medicine: Using Traditional Chinese Medicine for Harmony of Mind and Body by Tom Williams (Paperback - May 25, 2003)

8. Chinese Herbal Medicine: Formulas and Strategies by Dan Bensky and Randall Barolet (Hardcover – May 1990)

9. Tongue Diagnosis in Chinese Medicine by   Giovanni Maciocia (Hardcover - Jun 1995)

10. The Practice of Chinese Medicine: The Treatment of Diseases with Acupuncture and Chinese Herbs by Giovanni Maciocia (Hardcover - Dec 12, 2007)

11. Chinese Herbal Medicine: Materia Medica, Third Edition by Dan Bensky, Steven Clavey, Erich Stoger, and Andrew Gamble (Hardcover - Sep 2004)

12. Chinese Medicine for Beginners: Use the Power of the Five Elements to Heal Body and Soul by Achim Eckert (Paperback - Oct 2, 1996)

Other Books By Benita And Jim

Renewal

Feeling stressed? Anxious? Nervous? Learn what behaviors can feed stress and how to change these behaviors to reduce it. Learn stress management and the best ways to deal with panic attacks. Find other resources to help you cope with anxiety.
ISBN # 978-1440413347

Put Your Weight Loss in Overdrive

Do you want to lose weight? Are you willing to eat healthier and make changes in your diet? If you are willing to follow our lead and replace your unhealthy diet with even some of the super foods we tell you about in this book, you will put your diet in overdrive. Weight loss will be a snap. We guarantee it. This book makes weight loss easy.   ISBN # 978-1440413320

Life Management

Are you organized? Then you aren't the person we're looking for. If you aren't as organized as you think you should be, this is the book for you. Say goodbye to clutter and let order reign. We provide clever home and family management tips.; time saving tips and more. Get help managing your life.   ISBN # 978-1440417458

You Want It When?

Are you a procrastinator? Do you put off doing things until just before they're due? Do you do your Christmas shopping on Christmas Eve? There is help for all of you right here. Learn how to break the procrastination habit. ISBN # 978-1440417067

ABC's of Goal Setting

Ever set goals and write them down? What happened? Did you reach any of them or did you give up before you got there? Supercharge your goal setting and get ready for that satisfaction that only comes after reaching one of your goals. This book makes goal setting easy. ISBN # 978-1440419183

How Toxic Are You?

Everyone is subjected to toxins everyday. Over 80,000 at last count. Living away from the larger cities helps but not as much as you think. There are toxins in our water, our food, and in our air. What can we do to be healthy and survive our toxic world? Does fasting or jogging help? Yes, but not enough – toxins bind to fat cells. If you are at all interesting in your and your families health, this is a must read!
ISBN # 978-140425590

Coming Soon!

You Were Born To Excel

This book is based on a series of classes we compiled back in June of 1998. The classes were called Human Excellence Engineering. The basic series consisted of six classes as presented in this book. Two to three weeks were spent on each class. An advanced series was planned and begun but never completed. The topics covered are: In chapter 1: New Thinking Skills; in chapter 2: Inside You; in chapter 3: Changing the Past; in chapter 4: A Brighter Today; in chapter 5: Feeling Good Again; and in chapter 6: The Future Begins Here. The classes and hence, the material in this book are a combination of NLP, Psychology and Shamanism. ISBN # (not yet assigned)

Personal Trance-formations

More than ever, researchers are concerned with the effects of mental and emotional states on an individuals health and with the possibility of treating the patient as an active and responsible participant in the healing process rather than as a passive recipient of either the disease or the cure. It is this emphasis that provides the basis for using a variety of techniques that enable non-medical persons to control pain perception and create their own response to illness. The mind plays a vital role in healing, more even than modern medicine has so far acknowledged. This guidebook to your inner world, the inner landscape of your soul, will help you connect with your most authentic feelings and thoughts. It contains a variety of techniques for dealing with this deep inner material. ISBN # (not yet assigned)

Approaching Wisdom

Storytelling is essential to the shaman's craft. There was more to the old tales than just a good yarn. Woven into the thrills and emotions were messages. The tales are the framework of the lore and the lore is a body of teachings and an essential part of the shaman's working life. Through lore we re- create the ancient strands of Otherworldly knowledge buried deep in our unconscious and bring them to the forefront of our conscious mind. We can then see them from a new perspective and apply them to life in our "everyday" world. This book recreates the shaman's storytelling as a quest for wisdom. In it we explore ways through story, myth and exercises to expand your sensory awareness, achieve internal union and contact your transpersonal self. This book provides tools, but the real exploration is up to you. ISBN # (not yet assigned)

The Castle of the Grail

The Quest for the Grail is not a fairy tale for children. It is a serious undertaking.

The journey is full of trials and tribulations. The inner landscape of the Quest is full of dark forests, winding paths, narrow places, bridges, gates and castles. It is a very confusing place for us because we start foolish and ignorant. We do not recognize our guide and are frightened of what we might find. We are tested severely and ruthlessly but with mercy. The Quest is about Self Transformation and personal liberation. There is a unifying principle at the heart of all of these ways of thought, which can only be grasped by symbols, analogies and myths. Jung explained this with his archetypes of the collective unconscious.
ISBN # (not yet assigned)

The Gold Mine in PLR.

What is PLR? How can it benefit you? P.L. and R. are the initial letters of Private Label Rights. PLR is merchandise or software, most of which is info or text based, customizable, and reusable as your own. The concept of PLR differs only slightly from having a ghostwriter. So if you have a website and need fresh content or are a writer and need fresh ideas - this book is a must have! ISBN # (not yet assigned)

Creativity

Would you like to be more creative? More intuitive? Would you like to learn creative problem solving? You can with the proper training. You probably already are intuitive and creative without realizing it.

This book will provide the training you need to handle anything life throws at you in a more creative way.
ISBN # (not yet assigned)

Never Pay for Computer Software Again

Would you like to get a totally free operating system for your PC? How about an office suite that is rated better than Microsoft Office without Microsoft's price tag? Would you like free Image manipulation (Graphics) software? Games, Productivity software, Business applications - and all for free? How about one of the best web browsers around? Interested? It's all explained right here in Never Pay for Computer Software Again. Interested? You should be.
ISBN # (not yet assigned)

Surviving Life

How do you stay cheerful in the face of adversity, loss of job, bankruptcy, taxes and all the other things that life can throw at you? ISBN # (not yet assigned)

Take Control (It's Your Book)

Covers everything the author needs to know about self publishing. Copyrights, ISBN numbers, writing software versus page layout software, cover design, book layout, POD versus conventional printing methods, marketing, distribution, advertising, etc.
ISBN # (not yet assigned)

The Family Book of Fairy Tales

Stories of Princes and Princess's, enchanted giants and mighty ogres, lions, tailors and onions collected from around the world and assembled in this book to amuse you and your children. Includes the following stories: Cinderella's Daughter, The Giant's Hand, The Prince and the Lions, The Three Buns, The Boyer's Bride, How the Sea Became Salt, The Captive Princess, The Enchanted Oranges, The Knight of the Onion Shield, The Trade That No One Knew and The Prince and The Tailor. ISBN # (not yet assigned)

Benita's Encyclopedia of Crystals and Stones

What gems, crystals or stones have healing properties? Which do not? Which stones would you use for High Blood Pressure? Which for blood disorders? Which stones would be more effective for sores and wounds? How would you use Calcite in healing? ISBN # (not yet assigned)

Handy Order Form

Fax orders: 520-297-1293. (Send this form)

Telephone orders: 520-297-1293 Have your credit card handy.

Email orders: Tranzform@Comcast.net <Attn. Orders>

Postal orders: Orders * 8571 N. Calle Tioga * Oro Valley, Az. 85704

Please send the following books, software or reports. I understand that I may return any of them for a full refund for any reason.

ISBN No. _____ Quantity ☐

Title: _____

ISBN No. _____ Quantity ☐

Title: _____

Name: _____

Address: _____

City: _____ State : _____ Zip: _____

Phone: _____

Email: _____

I would like more information on other books and/ or

products _____ ☐

Arizona residents please add 8.1% Sales tax.

Handy Order Form

Fax orders: 520-297-1293. (Send this form)

Telephone orders: 520-297-1293 Have your credit card handy.

Email orders: Tranzform@Comcast.net <Attn. Orders>

Postal orders: Orders * 8571 N. Calle Tioga * Oro Valley, Az. 85704

Please send the following books, software or reports. I understand that I may return any of them for a full refund for any reason.

ISBN No. _____ Quantity ☐

Title: _____

ISBN No. _____ Quantity ☐

Title: _____

Name: _____

Address: _____

City: _____ State : _____ Zip: _____

Phone: _____

Email: _____

I would like more information on other books and/ or products _____ ☐

Arizona residents please add 8.1% Sales tax.

www.ingramcontent.com/pod-product-compliance
Lightning Source LLC
Chambersburg PA
CBHW071236170526
45165CB00003B/1126